Quit
Sugar
Quick

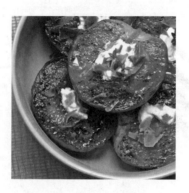

Jess Lomas

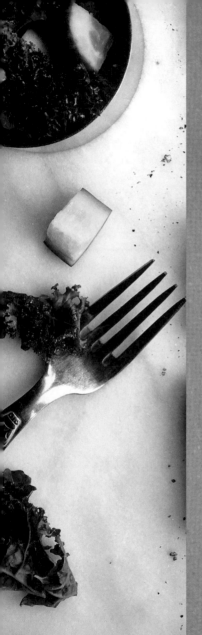

Published by:
Wilkinson Publishing Pty Ltd
ACN 006 042 173
Level 4, 2 Collins St Melbourne, Victoria,
Australia 3000
Ph: +61 3 9654 5446
www.wilkinsonpublishing.com.au

International distribution by Pineapple Media Limited
(www.pineapple-media.com)   ISSN 2203 9295

National Library of Australia Cataloguing-in-Publication entry:

Author: Lomas, Jess, author.

Title: Quit sugar quick / Jess Lomas.

ISBN: 9781922178671 (paperback)

Subjects: Sugar–Health aspects.
                 Food–Sugar content.
                 Sugar-free diet.
                 Sugar-free diet–Recipes.

Dewey Number   613.28332

Layout Design: Tango Media Pty Ltd

Cover Design: Tango Media Pty Ltd

Photos by agreement with iStock. Recipe photography
by agreement with Jess Lomas.

Printed in China

CONTENTS

HOW I
QUIT SUGAR QUICK

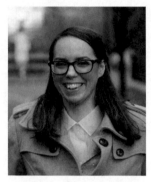

For many people, they can remember the specific moment in time when they knew that something in their life had to change and that after all the talking it was finally time to take action.

For years I had been aware that my diet contained too much added sugar, but like a lot of people I continued to battle on through the sweet highs, the depressing lows, the lethargy, lowered immunity, bad skin, and impaired concentration, amongst other symptoms.

I was fed up with constantly feeling unwell, and tired of how I felt within myself but it was the diagnosis of a close family member with type 2 diabetes that was my real wake up call. I knew then that I had to take responsibility for my own health, that I could get away with what I was doing for now, but that I would pay the price somewhere down the line.

I devised my own quit plan and decided to go cold turkey, dropping all refined sugar from my diet from a set date. The detox period made me realise I had been addicted to sugar, barely making it a day over the last decade without some form of added refined sugar sneaking its way into my diet.

There were plenty of moments of temptation during my first 30 days but I had made a commitment and was sticking to it for the sake of my health. I've put together *Quit Sugar Quick* from my experiences, knowing that it can be a daunting prospect to say no to refined sugar for 30 days, or consider giving it up for even longer.

Now, years after my sugar D-Day, I continue my re-education about the physiological and psychological effects of different foods on our bodies. Every new piece of information I learn, combined with how I feel when I wake up each day, reaffirms that my body, and your body, were not designed to consume the vast amounts of processed and sugary foods that have crept into the average diet.

The decision to change your lifestyle is a quick one, the commitment it takes to maintain it stretches a lifetime. From the other side of the sugar haze I can tell you with certainty, life with less sugar is most definitely sweeter.

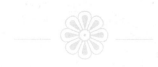

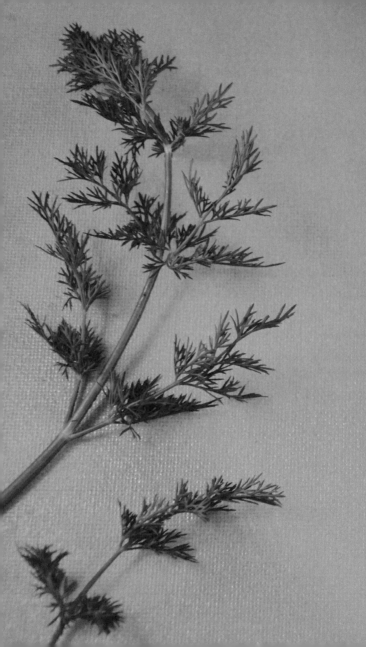

INTRODUCTION

It's undeniable that a low or no sugar diet is the latest trend in lifestyle and dieting. There has been an extraordinary influx of sugar free books, blogs and news articles over the last two years promoting the benefits of reducing the amount of refined sugar we consume.

From boasting increased energy and immunity to clearer skin and weight loss, it seems obvious to many that ditching the white stuff has many advantages. The old message that saturated fats are the cause of our increasing rates of overweight, obesity, diabetes and heart disease is out, and the new truth is that highly processed foods packed with excess fructose are the real enemy.

In 2014, the World Heath Organization (WHO) confirmed what several sugar-free advocates had been saying for years when they revived the debate over recommended daily allowances for added sugar in the diet. From a previously recommended 10%, the WHO began advising that no more than 5% of a person's diet should be made up of added sugars, to reduce the risk of developing diseases such as diabetes.

These added sugars come from convenience and takeaway products, pre-packaged foods including sauces, dressings, spreads, pre-marinated meat, low-fat products including dairy, and bread products. These are classed as "hidden sugars", meaning many people do not realise there is sugar lurking in the often long list of ingredients. Why would a box of breakfast cereal need 36.5 grams of sugar per 100 grams? Why would a bottle of low-fat salad dressing need 22.3 grams of sugar per

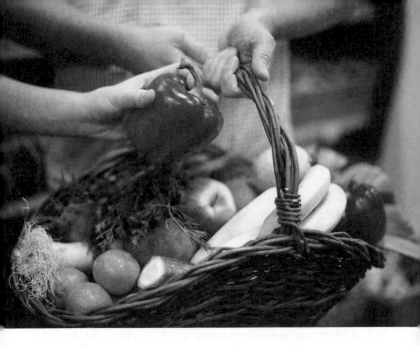

100 grams, or a bottle of tomato sauce need 29 grams of sugar per 100 grams?

It's the food industry's dirty little secret that isn't so secret anymore; add sugar to your product and you not only increase its shelf life but you also hook your customers in to the irresistible taste, ensuring they come back for more. Sugar is also a relatively cheap ingredient, especially in the age of high fructose corn syrup, and so from an economic perspective, it makes sense why products pumped full of sweeteners are so affordable to both the manufacturers and the consumers.

The other type of added sugars invading our diets are "known sugars", which make up products we already associate as being sweet and perhaps unhealthy, such as fruit juices, sodas, chocolate bars, cakes and other desserts. These "treats" have become daily occurrences for a large percentage of the population and are no longer an infrequent event. We know they're not the healthiest option but more often than not we can't resist that orange juice with breakfast, muffin for morning tea, soda with lunch or chocolate biscuit after dinner.

When you add up the known and unknown sugars we consume daily it can amount to a frightening level that our bodies struggle to process. For the majority, in only a couple of generations we've moved from home grown and home cooked meals to total dependence on supermarkets and corporations to fill our shopping trolleys and stomachs. We often don't question whether a product is safe or not due to a naïve belief that if it exists on a supermarket shelf it can't be overly harmful to us; surely it's passed a long list of tests and guidelines to get there, even if we can't recognise or understand the complex list of ingredients on the label.

From time to time, eating packaged foods is unavoidable, and to be fair can even be enjoyable. Re-evaluating the amount of sugar in your diet is not a punishment, and guides such as *Quit Sugar Quick* do not exist to deprive you of the finer things in life. Reducing the amount of added sugar in your diet is a lifelong journey with ups and downs, but to start it only takes a 30 day commitment.

You make a choice every time you eat a meal, visit a supermarket or dine at a restaurant, will you be fuelling your

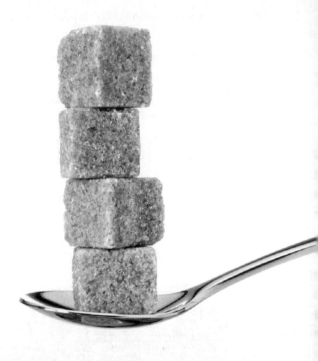

When you add up the known and unknown sugars we consume daily it can amount to a frightening level that our bodies struggle to process.

body or feeding its addictions? Salt, sugar and fat are the three tastes our bodies go wild for; the more you eat the more you crave. In order to break this cycle you need to break the habit and realign your tastebuds, emotions and mind.

In only 30 days you can reset your body to recognise and appreciate the natural sweetness in foods, and reject the abundance of added sweetness that has crept into our lives. It's an interesting ride I can assure you, there'll be good days and bad, and at the end of the month you'll know one way or another where you personally stand with sugar.

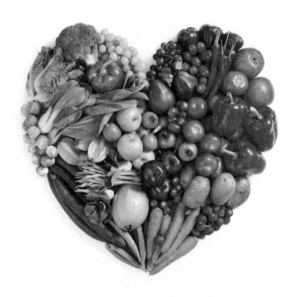

Salt, sugar and fat are the three tastes our bodies go wild for; the more you eat the more you crave. In order to break this cycle you need to break the habit and realign your tastebuds, emotions and mind.

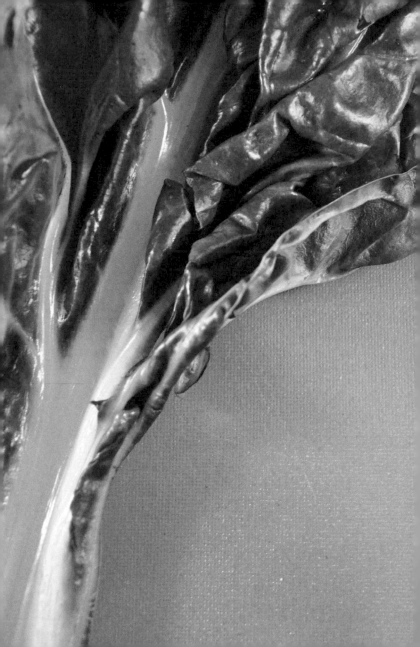

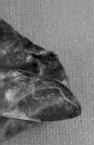

WHY SUGAR?

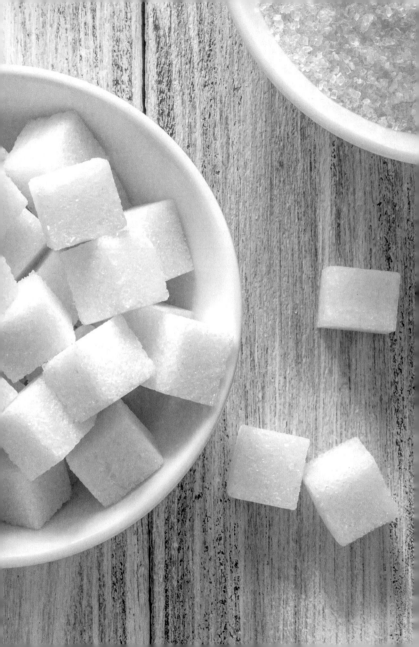

B efore you start on your journey it's important to know why. When we point the finger of shame at sugar it is fructose we are specifically talking about. Fructose is a simple sugar that our body uses for energy, along with glucose. In small amounts, found in whole fruits and vegetables, the body processes fructose effectively as the fibre content of these foods slows down the absorption rate. Once you add increased amounts of fructose, and at multiple intervals during the day, the body begins to struggle.

When you eat carbohydrates your body releases insulin to extract the glucose to fuel your system. The liver only processes approximately 20% of this thanks to an in-built mechanism that prohibits it from absorbing too much. When fructose is consumed in large quantities (such as in a large glass or two of soda or fruit juice) it is poorly digested by the gastrointestinal tract and heads straight to the liver; it's almost as if it's invisible to the body. Your liver then works hard to process the fructose, the at-times toxic load putting this vital organ under immense strain.

Too much fructose equals an overworked liver and excess fatty acids and fat in the system, and can lead to a multitude of issues including diabetes, heart disease, insulin resistance and fatty liver disease. Most commonly the excess fructose manifests itself as weight gain, sluggishness and lowered immunity. This is an extremely simplified explanation of why fructose is wreaking havoc on our bodies but for most people this is all they need to begin reevaluating how they feel.

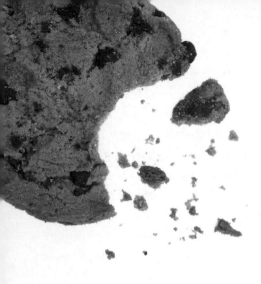

Sugar is an addiction that starts young and stays with us throughout our life, whether we want to acknowledge it or not. What has taken so long to build cannot be demolished in a matter of days or weeks but takes time, patience, perseverance, commitment and courage.

Too much fructose equals an overworked liver and excess fatty acids and fat in the system, and can lead to a multitude of issues including diabetes, heart disease, insulin resistance and fatty liver disease.

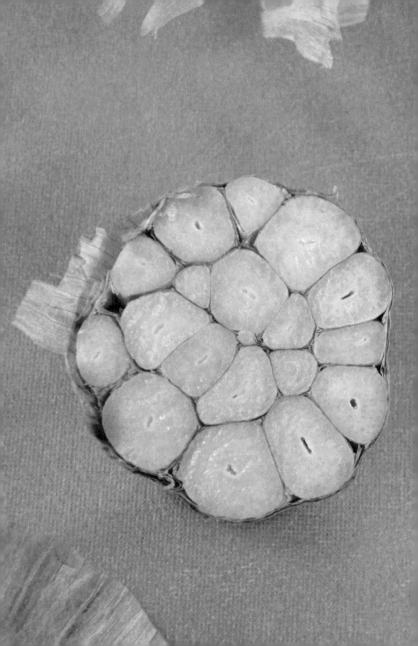

QUICK SUGAR QUESTIONS

HOW MUCH FRUCTOSE CAN I EAT A DAY?

As advised by the American Heart Association, men should have no more than 36 grams (9 teaspoons) of added sugar daily; women no more than 20 grams (5 teaspoons) and children 12 grams (3 teaspoons).

CAN I EAT FRUIT?

The body can easily process the amount of fructose in two pieces of fruit a day. Fruit should not be excluded from your regular diet unless you want to, in which case it's important to increase your vegetable consumption. Aim to include more berries, eat fruit whole with its skin, and avoid fruit juice, even home squeezed. Fruit juice ranks as high on the fructose scale as some sodas and is no substitute for a glass of water. If making your own juice at home, stick to the 80-20 rule: 80% vegetables and 20% fruit, usually half an apple can suffice to provide enough sweetness.

CAN I EAT DRIED FRUIT?

As fruit is dried it is dehydrated of the majority of its water content, this is great for preserving a food but in doing so the sugar content increases. Also, as the fruit is dehydrated its size decreases, meaning you can eat more without filling up as quickly, and you end up ingesting more sugar. Be mindful of adding dried fruit to breakfast muesli, in trail mixes (unless you are actually going hiking and require the sugar hit) and in school lunches for the kids, eat the whole fruit instead.

WHAT IS THE FRUCTOSE CONTENT OF SOME COMMON FRUITS?

Lemon (1 medium) – 0.6 grams

Raspberries (1 cup) – 3 grams

Kiwifruit (1 medium) – 3.4 grams

Strawberries (1 cup) – 3.8 grams

Grapefruit (1/2 medium) – 4.3 grams

Orange (1 medium) – 6.1 grams

Banana (1 medium) – 7.1 grams

Apple (1 medium) – 9.5 grams

Raisins (1/4 cup) – 12.3 grams

Dried apricots (1 cup) – 16.4 grams

Dried figs (1 cup) – 23 grams

The Sugar Fix: The High Fructose Fallout that is Making You Fat and Sick, Richard Johnson and Timothy Cower, Gallery Books, 2009.

CAN I EAT HONEY AND MAPLE SYRUP?

Locally sourced raw honey that hasn't been heat-treated has an abundance of healing properties to consider beyond its fructose content. You won't find this type of honey on your supermarket shelf, anything sitting there has been treated and processed to remove all of the beneficial elements and leave only the sweetness. Your local farmer's market is a great source for raw honey, as is the Internet. Raw honey ensures a premium product that has retained most or all of the beneficial enzymes, natural vitamins and antioxidants. It is anti viral, anti bacterial, promotes good digestive health and can be a powerful aid in treating allergies, particularly hay fever. A little bit goes a long way so you'll find a jar of raw honey will keep you going for many months, if not longer. If you can't source good quality raw honey don't substitute with a supermarket shelf brand, simply avoid it entirely.

As with honey, maple syrup comes in myriad of qualities and the more you pay, the purer the product will be. It is incredibly sweet so a small amount goes a long way. Its health benefits include a high level of manganese, which is great for energy and in strengthening your immunity, and high levels of zinc, also good for the immune system and for reproductive health. Look for organic Grade A pure maple syrup and avoid maple "flavoured" syrup, which is a highly refined product lacking the benefits of the pure product.

CAN I DRINK ALCOHOL?

Yes ... and no. While moderation is the key, not all alcohol is created equal when it comes to fructose levels. Red wine, beer and straight spirits including gin, vodka and whisky are safer options but leave the mixer drinks such as cola, fruit juice and tonic water out of your glass.

The level of fructose in winemaking grapes has decreased significantly by the time you drink the final product thanks to the process of fermentation. While white wine undergoes this same process it still retains more sugar than red, with dessert wines and champagne joining it on the less than desirable but okay sometimes list. The sugar in beer is maltose, not fructose, and so is okay to drink, in moderation.

WHAT ARE SOME SAFER SUGAR ALTERNATIVES TO USE?

In addition to raw honey and Grade A maple syrup, stevia and rice malt syrup are two easy sugar alternatives that you can usually find in your local supermarket. Each has both positive and negative aspects to its use. Fruit also makes a great sweetener. It's important when removing excess sugar from your diet not to simply replace white or brown sugar with a "safe" sugar alternative. It is far better to remove the craving for or habit of consuming sweetened foods outside of fruit and vegetables.

Stevia is a plant-derived granulated sweetener gaining favour around the world. The danger with stevia is that it is up to 200 times sweeter than white sugar so it's not as simple as a 1:1 substitute. Depending on the brand used, some stevia can also leave a bitter aftertaste that may put some people off using it again. The other downside to using stevia is the price;

while it's more readily available on supermarket shelves, the price is not relative to white sugar and may not be a viable alternative for those on a budget.

Rice malt syrup is a complex carbohydrate with maltose (malt sugar) and a small amount of glucose. It can usually be found in the health food aisle of most supermarkets or from health food stores or online. It is relatively cheap and a little tends to go a long way but being a liquid is not as easy to substitute in recipes calling for granulated sugar and may take some experimenting to perfect. It's important when buying rice malt syrup to check the ingredients list contains 100% rice and no additives, preservatives or fillers.

The recipes in *Quit Sugar Quick* use fruit and rice malt syrup for sweetening if necessary. You may want to experiment with stevia, just remember to significantly decrease the amount you use.

WHAT SUGAR ALTERNATIVES ARE BEST AVOIDED?

Artificial sweeteners such as aspartame, often used in diet soft drinks, are manufactured, heavily processed and not recommended. Aspartame is often used in "low sugar" or "sugar free" products including cookies and desserts. While research into the effects of aspartame is ongoing, negative health effects are thought to include increased risk of cancer. Other fake sugars to avoid include sucralose, saccharine and

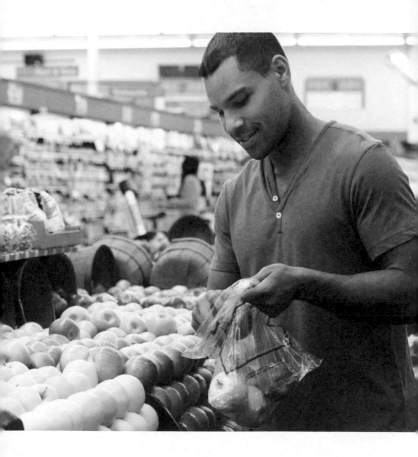

alcohol-based sweeteners such as sorbitol. When choosing a
sweetener, fructose is a consideration but it is far better to
use a smaller amount of a whole foods sweetener such as raw
honey or a couple of dates than to use larger amounts of an
artificial sweetener such as aspartame.

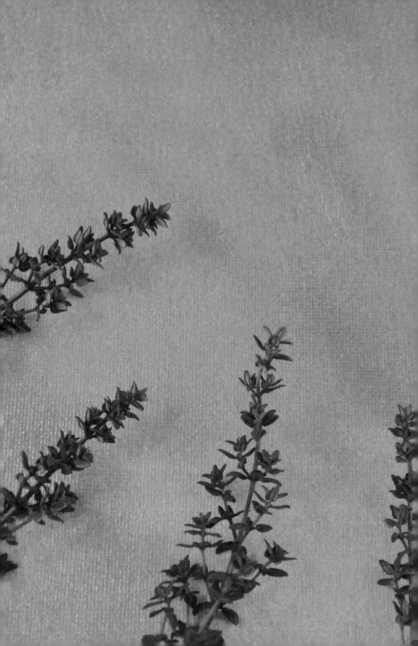

QUIT SUGAR QUICK
ACTION PLAN

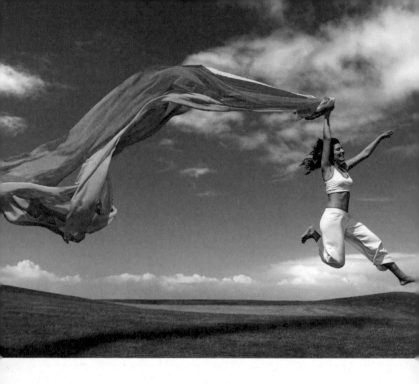

Making the decision to become more conscious of what you eat and reducing your sugar intake is a lifestyle change and a lifelong journey, not a diet. It may sound clichéd but you must take each day as it comes, ride out the missteps and less than ideal choices, and congratulate yourself regularly for investing in your health and happiness.

Your motto going forward is to remove the everyday excesses and enjoy the occasional sweetness in life. Making the decision to prioritise your health is a great start but there are hard days ahead, I won't sugarcoat it (pun intended). As you detox your body of its sugar dependence, some people may suffer from withdrawal symptoms, some may "relapse" before their detox is complete, and a lucky few will sail through relatively unscathed.

There are many schools of thought about how long the detox process takes; it's different for each person, but what those numbers represent is a goal because without a goal you will never know when you've reached a milestone.

To achieve the goal of reducing excess sugar in your diet I recommend the 30-30 rule. The 30-30 rule is simple, and is in fact not a rule but a sign post to mark your progress. Aim for 30 days of mindful, low sugar eating and when day 30 draws to a close, look ahead to the following 30 days. Taking this journey one month at a time makes it more achievable than an open-ended time period that doesn't allow for special occasions or holidays. For some people 30 days will be long enough to change old habits and thinking, while others may have to look beyond one or two months until they feel in control of their cravings.

Of course there's a bit more to cutting out sugar than setting a 30-day goal, so keep reading.

DO YOUR RESEARCH

Take some time before D-Day to read a variety of opinions on low-fructose or fructose-free living. The more you read, the easier it will be to decide where you sit; will you give sugar up entirely or just reduce processed foods and refined sugar in your diet?

Making the decision to become more conscious of what you eat and reducing your sugar intake is a lifestyle change and a lifelong journey, not a diet.

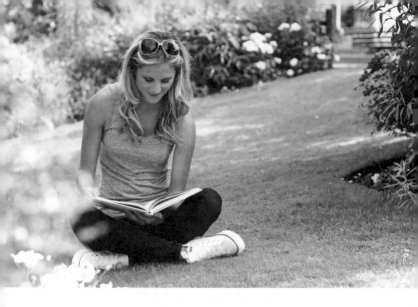

Utilise the Internet and spend some time reading sugar-free blogs that offer testimonials of other people's journey; save any recipes that catch your eye to a folder for later use, cross-check facts and opinions, and make use of the online community, whether through blogs or Facebook groups who are there to support each other.

COMMIT

Now that you know why you're kicking sugar to the curb, it's time to commit. It's easy to tell yourself, and even others, that you "need" to stop eating so much sugar but it's harder to actually follow through with it. It's now time for you to share your commitment with someone close to you, such as a partner, family member or friend. In essence, **sharing your commitment** makes you accountable and will help you stick to your new lifestyle by having someone to reach out to when times get tough. Through sharing with friends or family, questions may be raised that you hadn't yet thought of; how will you handle this temptation? What will you do if something unexpected happens? Now is a good time to get a second, third or fourth opinion before you dive in.

If you don't feel comfortable sharing your commitment with anyone just yet, commit to yourself and write a letter. **Explain** why you are making this decision, how you felt before starting your journey, and how you hope to feel after the first 30, 60 and 90 days. You might like to plan how you will tackle difficult situations like birthdays and holidays; will you embrace the spirit of the occasion and enjoy a piece of cake, or will you politely decline? Writing a letter is a great way to remind yourself down the track why you started this; you could even keep a journal as you go to look back at how far you've come.

THE LAST HURRAH!

Some people may want to skip this step, in fact there's little sense and definitely no science to stuffing your face with as much sugar as possible but for some people, such as myself, this was the final nail in the coffin for ditching the white stuff.

Set a start date for your Quit Sugar Quick journey. I chose the week after Easter and gave myself Easter Sunday to indulge

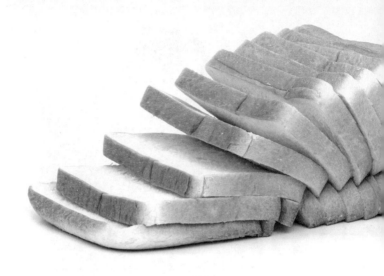

in what, at the time, I had convinced myself I would miss. It was a sugar cocktail that made me feel ill almost instantly. It's the perfect activity for reminding you why you are about to take on an incredible detox, but if you're ready now, skip this step and move onto the cleanse.

Your last hurrah may take on other forms, from sitting down with your favourite block of chocolate to going out to a special restaurant and sampling a couple of desserts, or it may be using a jar of sauce or dressing you know is chock-full of excess sugar, salt and other less desirables. Your last hurrah, like the rest of this journey, is **unique to you**. Set a date, indulge (or don't) and enjoy, then get ready for the next step.

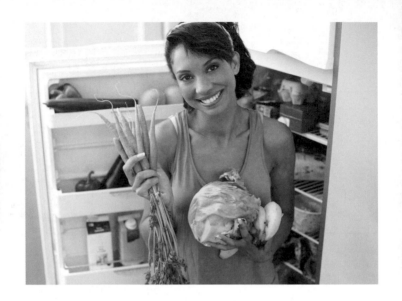

CLEANSE THE HOUSE

Despite how it sounds, this doesn't involve a traditional smoke ceremony or getting in an expert to check the Feng Shui of your rooms. Cleansing your house begins and ends in your kitchen. Set aside a period of time where you can pull everything out of the cupboards and refrigerator. Read the nutritional labels and decide if it's a keeper or headed for the bin.

Start with the cupboards then move on to the refrigerator and freezer; remove any sauces, dressings, frozen desserts and ready-made meals. Those with a waste not-want not mindset might like to donate the discarded items to a family member or friend who hasn't decided to join you on your adventure.

Despite how it sounds, this doesn't involve a traditional smoke ceremony or getting in an expert to check the Feng Shui of your rooms. Cleansing your house begins and ends in your kitchen.

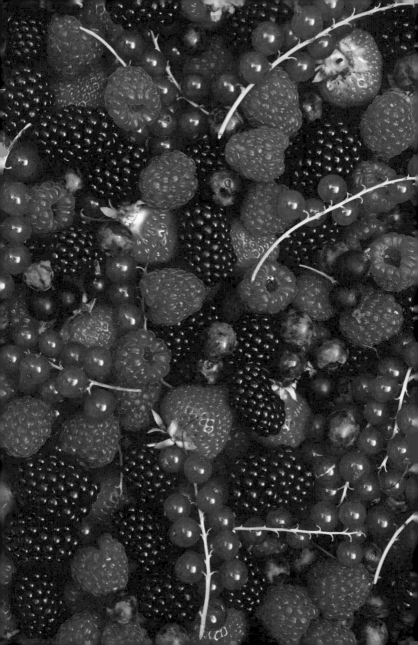

Now that you've cleaned out the old it's important to **introduce the new**; head to your local supermarket or fresh food store and stock up on fresh vegetables, protein-rich meat, free-range eggs, good fats such as avocados, spices, nuts and seeds. When you begin your detox you might have cravings that urge you to reach for something sweet and by stocking your home with healthy options you're helping future you out of a sticky situation.

At this point it's best to **remove fruit** from your shopping list, it can be reintroduced after the first 30 days. It's important to abstain from anything overly sweet, even unrefined fructose in fruit, for at least the first two weeks as your body goes through detox. You'll be surprised when you take your first bite of an apple after detox at **just how sweet it is**, and in turn you might find you now need a smaller amount to satiate your appetite. Don't worry about missing out on the healthy benefits of whole fruit; by increasing your vegetable intake and diversifying the types of vegetables you eat you'll have all your vitamin and mineral bases covered.

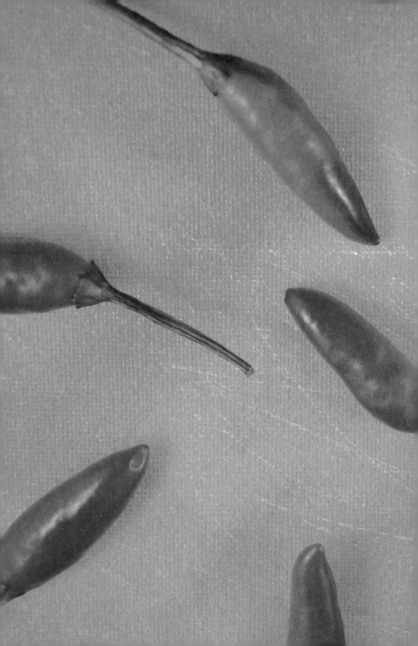

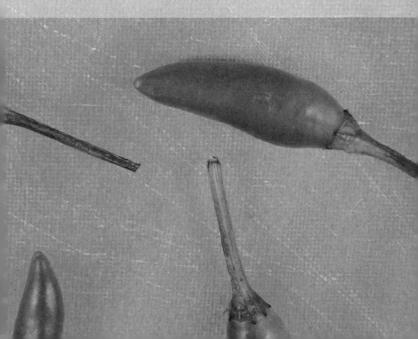

LET'S GET STARTED

You've decided to lower or quit your sugar intake, you've read a few books or online articles, have an idea of how far you want to take it, have committed to doing it either just to yourself or to a friend or loved one, have cleansed your kitchen of sugary and processed foods … now what?

Take your Quit Sugar Quick journey **one day at a time**. Focus first on changing your habits and loving yourself through the detox. Next, concentrate on whole food nutrition and cooking from scratch, and don't forget to keep checking your progress as you go.

Remember to aim for the 30-30 rule, 30 days of mindful, low sugar eating before stopping to evaluate your progress, congratulate yourself on your achievements and look ahead to the coming 30 days. Break this down from week to week to make it easier.

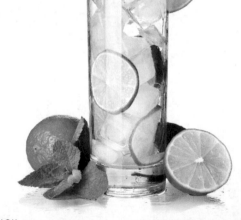

WEEK ONE

Begin to change your habits

You've removed any high sugar products from your cupboards and have restocked your refrigerator with fresh, whole food ingredients, but once you leave your home you come face to face with a world of temptation. There's convenience stores to duck into for a quick sugar fix, someone's birthday at the office, an afternoon tea out with friends, or a work dinner that can't be avoided; these are scenarios you will continually face so it's time to work out your battle plan now.

The earlier you learn to say no to sugar, the easier the first 30 days will be. Week One is a great time to start substituting old sugar habits with new, healthier ones. Replace breakfast cereal with eggs served on steamed spinach, replace the lunchtime can of soda with a carbonated water, and take a platter of cheese into the office for a colleague's birthday in addition to the birthday cake, offering those without a sweet tooth an alternative. It's all about creative thinking to get out of old patterns and habits.

Avoid swapping to a lesser-of-the-two-evils option, even if it is only temporary. If soda is your Achilles' heel, try cutting back by 50% during the first week and drinking sparkling water in between, rather than switching over to the aspartame-sweetened "diet" beverages. If drinking coffee or tea is unbearable without a little sugar, try to reduce the amount you

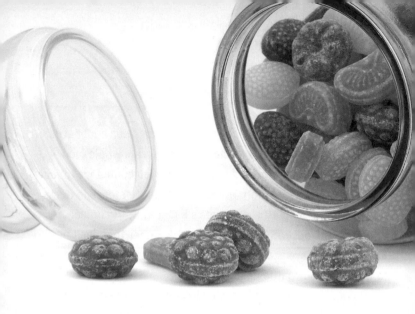

add. The ideal resolution is to enjoy your beverages au naturel and sweetener free but for now reduce the added sugar to your drinks by half and aim for zero added sweeteners by the start of Week Two.

By the end of Week One you may not have experienced any substantial withdrawal symptoms beyond the odd craving or two. This will of course depend on how much sugar you used to eat, and in what forms, highly processed and "obvious" sugars (such as in soda and desserts) or "hidden" sugars in pre-packaged products, dried fruit or fruit juice.

If you've already experienced cravings, the best way to banish them is to eat a **protein rich snack** or meal and drink a glass of water, or try some of the tips to beat cravings from page 60.

Often a Week One craving is emotional or mental rather than an actual physical craving, which will come later in Week Two. You're so used to eating or drinking a certain something that the break in habit causes you to think about eating or drinking that thing more frequently than usual. By actively eating something that will fill you up, you squash the craving in its tracks before your brain can try and convince you to give in.

Week One Tips

1. Substitute old habits for new, healthier ones.

2. Replace soda with carbonated water.

3. Cut down or go cold turkey, it's up to you. Either reduce the frequency of sugary foods, aiming to get down to zero servings by the start of Week Two, or eliminate sugar entirely from day one.

4. If you're experiencing cravings, eat a protein rich snack or drink a glass of water.

WEEK TWO

Love yourself

The first two weeks of a sugar detox will be the hardest as your body nudges you at every opportunity to eat something sweet; Week Two is the time to stick to your guns and ride the detox wave. Symptoms you may experience include headaches, body aches and sweats, interrupted sleep, nausea and overwhelming cravings. You may experience none, some or all of these.

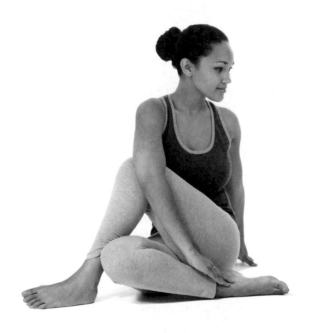

It's important during Week One and Two to make time to relax. Try not to do any extreme exercise but stick to **low impact activities** such as yoga, walking or swimming. Your body will be going through a large change and it's likely you won't be feeling at your peak during this time, so there's no need to add extra stress by attempting to learn rock climbing now or entering yourself in a marathon. Equally, this is not a time to sit and do nothing, waiting for the cravings to overwhelm you. Going for a gentle walk is a great way to stave off any cravings as well as clear your head.

If possible during Week Two, make an appointment for a massage or facial, some activity where you can be pampered and where the toxins leaving your system can have a helping hand. Having a sauna or sitting in a steam room is also great for both relaxation and toxin release, just remember to **rehydrate** during and afterwards.

Loving yourself can also mean going to see a movie, taking time to finish reading a book, going on a date night, booking a weekend away, anything that nurtures your soul.

Week Two will be the hardest physically so it's important to remember to love and **be kind to yourself** during this time. Work may be unavoidable, but keep your weeknights free of social activity unless absolutely necessary. Your energy levels may be low, and physically you may start to feel like you're coming down with a cold. Putting unnecessary stress on your system by still trying to do it all and see everyone will only make Week Two more miserable for you.

By now you should have zero added sugar in your diet; sodas and fruit juices should be replaced with carbonated or plain water, coffee and tea should be without sugar or not drunk at all. You should be restricting both known sugars, such as chocolate, as well as hidden sugars, such as flavoured yoghurts, dressings and sauces. You should also be focusing on increasing your vegetable intake by aiming to eat something green with every meal.

Week Two Tips

1. Your diet should now include no added sugar; it's time to face the detox head on.

2. Try not to eat any fruit from now until the end of the 30 days to realign your taste buds.

3. Above all remember to love yourself; this is a special week to nurture your body through the withdrawal symptoms.

4. If possible book in a massage or facial, or have a sauna or foot spa to help eliminate toxins and ease the withdrawal process.

Loving yourself can also mean going to see a movie, taking time to finish reading a book, going on a date night, booking a weekend away, anything that nurtures your soul.

WEEK THREE

Eat to live

How are you feeling? Hopefully by the beginning of Week Three you're starting to feel more like yourself again, or perhaps starting to feel like a new person. By now the withdrawal symptoms should be subsiding, but don't be surprised if they linger a little longer; continue to be **gentle on yourself** and take time out of every day to relax.

As Week Three begins you can start increasing your activity level, perhaps booking in a game of tennis with friends or increasing the length of your workouts. You should start to feel a **renewed energy** with all the whole foods you've been eating. Your body may have gone through a period of shock as it waited day in day out for the usual fructose fix, but by now it's caught on to your new lifestyle and the foggy, listless you of two weeks ago should be a distant memory. Don't worry if this doesn't quite sound like how you're feeling, it's different for everyone and it may take you a bit more time to start feeling better.

Week Three is all about **eating to live**. When you reduce the amount of excess fructose in your diet, you release the body's natural ability to regulate its appetite. You may have asked yourself why it is you fill up so easily eating a big steak or even cheese and crackers compared to a packet of cookies that may disappear easily in one sitting. You don't fill up because the body's three appetite hormones, insulin, leptin and

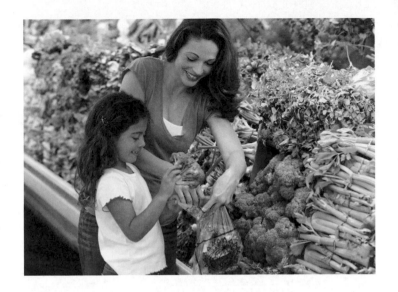

cholecystokinin don't respond when a flood of fructose comes in, and so you keep eating more and more. Once you reduce your fructose intake, you'll find yourself more aware of true hunger as well as finding you feel full from eating less food.

By reducing excess sugar in your diet you're not filling up on empty calories and you're truly eating to live. By forcing yourself to **prepare meals from scratch** it's likely you've gone for simpler meals that require fewer ingredients and don't take long to cook, or you're following the 7-day meal plan provided at the back of this book. The good news is now that you're realigning your taste buds to appreciate the abundant flavours in all foods, and not just sweet foods, a simple meal delivers the same satisfaction as a more elaborate recipe.

Focus on food in Week Three. Start a recipe folder and add recipes you might like to try; if they include fruit or alternative sweeteners, save these for after the first 60 days of low fructose eating. Spend a little extra time at the supermarket, greengrocer or farmer's market this week getting to know some vegetables you may not have tried before. Speak to the shop assistant and ask questions about how to store and prepare the vegetable, you'll be surprised at the knowledge they'll have to impart. The same applies for your local butcher or fishmonger, if you haven't spoken to them before, now is the time to strike up a relationship, ask about cuts of meat or specials.

Week Three Tips

1. Increase activity this week if you feel up to it.

2. Start a recipe folder of low fructose recipes to try.

3. Focus on food – speak to your local greengrocer about their produce.

4. Try a new vegetable this week.

WEEK FOUR

Check your progress

You can see the finish line on the horizon, you're almost there! Thirty days seemed like a long time back when you began your journey but you're about to reach the end, so it's time to check your progress and reflect on how you went, congratulate yourself on this incredible achievement, and look ahead to the next 30 days.

Take some time this week to sit down and think or write about how you found the first 30 day experience. Focus on one bad experience and one positive; it may have been a time you gave in to a craving or you may have thought negatively about yourself and your progress. Think about the bad experience first and how you might avoid repeating it in your upcoming 30 days. Was it a temptation that you know can be avoided next time? Can you now detect the warning signs that might lead to you thinking negatively about your progress? Was it a particular person that helped stir up these feelings? Can you talk to them about it? Make a resolution about how to deal with the issue if it arises again.

Now let go of the negative and move on to the positive experience, hopefully there will be more than one you can call upon. Why was this moment great? Did you navigate a week of birthday parties without touching a slice of cake? Did you manage to wean yourself off your soda addiction? Did you wake

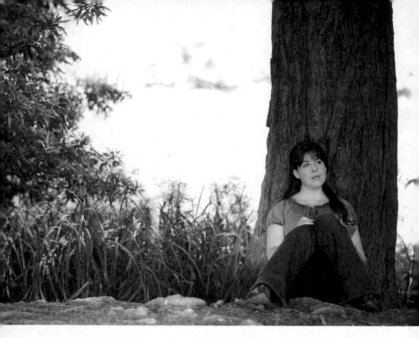

up one day feeling happy within yourself? Whatever it was that stood out to you about the last 30 days, take some time to enjoy it all over again. These are the moments that will provide fuel for you to keep going into the next 30 days and beyond and can be called upon when your next craving hits or when you begin to doubt your motivation or progress.

This last week is for reflecting on what worked and didn't work for you, your strengths and weaknesses, and how you can know and understand them better to help you over the next 30 days. Being honest with yourself at this point is crucial.

At the end of Week Four you can reintroduce fruit into your diet if you feel like it. It's good to start with berries and work your way from there, perhaps try adding them to your breakfast to begin with. If you removed fruit by the end of Week One at the latest, you might be surprised by how sweet it tastes now. Be careful not to fall back into old habits and let fruit be your gateway to sweeter things; stick to **one serving of fruit a day** for the next 30 days before returning to two servings a day after that.

Week Four Tips

1. Sit down and evaluate your first 30 days, what worked and didn't work.

2. Choose one negative and one positive experience to learn from and to call upon to get you through the next 30 days.

3. Slowly begin to reintroduce fruit by the end of the week, stick to one serving for the next 30 days before returning to two if desired.

4. Congratulate yourself for an incredible achievement – 30 days into your new lifestyle!

5. Look ahead to the next 30 days.

REPEAT

Once you've reflected on the past 30 days, taken time to revel in your success and celebrated your achievements, it's time to look forward to the next 30 days. Thirty days is only one month to change your life, and as one month draws to a close it's time to get ready for the next.

You may still be struggling with your sweet tooth, with saying no to sugar or dealing with the lingering detox symptoms, be assured that the next 30 days will be easier, there's no looking back!

The good news as you enter your second block of 30 days is that you won't have to deal with excessive withdrawal symptoms, the detox is done! Keep up the home cooked meals using whole food ingredients, avoid processed food, utilise supplements to suppress cravings (see page 60), try eating a green vegetable with every meal, do some form of exercise or movement every day, and keep educating yourself. When looking for tips to get through the second block of 30 days, look to Week Three and Week Four for guidance; you've done the hard yards and thrown sugar to the curb, now it's about being vigilant and not reintroducing it. If you stumble from time to time don't criticise yourself, nobody is perfect and tomorrow is a new day.

At the end of the second block of 30 days (Week Eight) it's time to increase your fruit to two servings a day, if you want. You may find that you're happy with your one serving or you might be eager to reintroduce more. It's also time to start considering sugar alternatives, such as raw honey, rice malt syrup or stevia for when you want a treat. I am not recommending you make a sweet treat a daily or weekly occurrence, or even force yourself to try a sweet recipe at this stage. That said, the treat recipes in *Quit Sugar Quick* use minimal sweetener, often relying on the natural sweetness of fruit for flavour.

Take your journey 30 days at a time: reduce or eliminate, stop and evaluate, congratulate and look forward to the next 30 days. Focus on feeding your body whole foods instead of processed foods, invest in your education by allocating time to reading books and articles or watching documentaries about food, get back in the kitchen and cook from scratch, love yourself through the positive moments and even more through the weaker times, and above all don't forget to enjoy life with the occasional treat if you choose to.

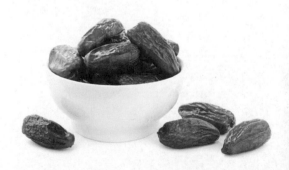

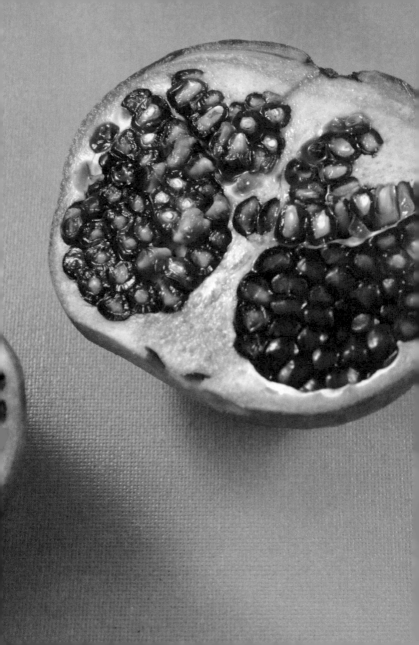

BEAT THE
CRAVINGS

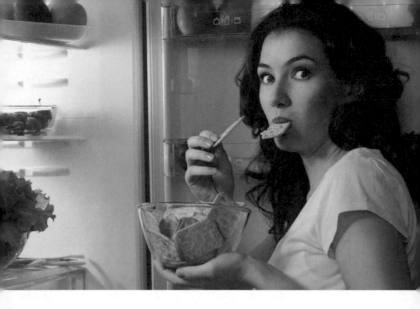

1. Eat more protein and good fats to fill you up.

2. Drink a glass of water; dehydration is often a hidden cause behind food cravings.

3. Take chromium supplements to help regulate blood sugar levels and ease sugar cravings. The recommended daily dose is 600-1,000mg a day, taken with food.

4. Magnesium is another supplement that helps regulate blood sugar and can ease sugar cravings; it also stabilises mood and emotions, helping you cope better with the stress of going through a major detox.

5. Snack on a sweeter vegetable such as a carrot to subdue your sugar craving.

6. Try yoga. According to yoga guru Tara Stiles, the best pose for a sugar craving is a seated meditation with arms in a "V" as it allows your mind to refocus. Maintain this pose for 3 minutes.

7. Distract yourself by doing a physical activity such as going for a walk or vacuuming the house.

8. Brush your teeth. It may seem like a strange tactic but it serves two purposes, sending a message to your brain that you have finished eating, and also distracting you from your cravings.

9. Clean up after dinner by washing dishes and packing any leftovers away. Remove food from sight to signal to your brain that eating time is over.

10. Move away from the television; mindless eating goes hand in hand with mindless entertainment.

11. To avoid late night cravings have a hot shower or bath to signal to your body you are preparing for sleep and not eating.

12. Remove the source; use willpower to not bring sugary foods home from the supermarket in the first place.

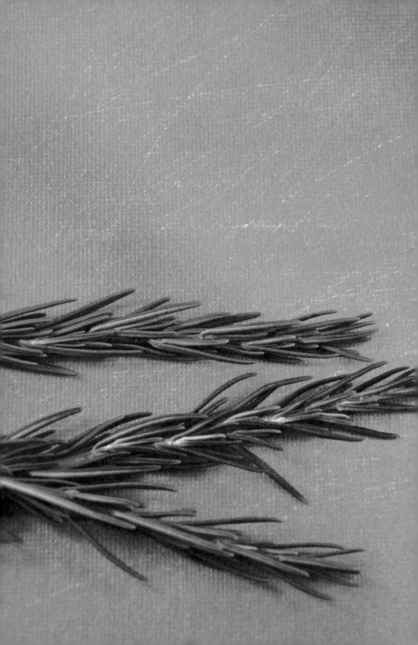

RECIPES

BREAKFAST

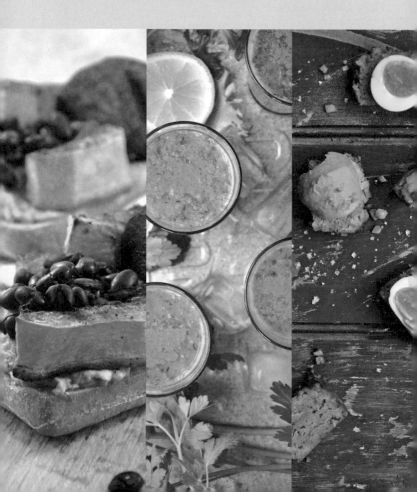

QUINOA VEGETABLE SCRAMBLE

AVOCADO & WHITE BEAN SMASH
ON ROASTED MUSHROOMS

ROASTED VEGETABLE FRITTATA

ONE PAN BREAKFAST

WAKE ME UP SMOOTHIE

SWEET POTATO AND BACON
MINI LOAVES

CHUNKY VEG BRUSCHETTA

Quinoa Vegetable Scramble

Serves 1

1 cup (approximately 200g) lightly steamed mixed vegetables of choice (e.g. broccoli & cauliflower florets, diced pumpkin, peas)

1 cup (180g) cooked quinoa
1½ tsp smoked paprika
1 tsp ground turmeric
½ tsp sea salt
2 eggs

1. Heat up a drizzle of extra virgin olive oil in a frying pan and add vegetables, quinoa and seasonings. Stir through until heated.

2. Crack the eggs into a small bowl and whisk until the yolk and white are just combined.

3. Add the eggs to the frying pan and use a spatula or spoon to work the egg mixture through the quinoa and vegetables until cooked to your liking.

4. Remove from the heat and serve with a sprinkling of finely chopped parsley if desired.

AVOCADO & WHITE BEAN SMASH ON ROASTED MUSHROOMS

Serves 1

1 cup (60g) small mushrooms
15g/1oz unsalted butter, melted
3 sprigs of fresh thyme
1 garlic clove, crushed
½ an avocado
½ cup (100g) cannellini beans (or any white bean)

¼ cup (60ml) fresh lemon juice
¼ cup (10g) flat leaf parsley, finely chopped
1 tsp chilli flakes (or fresh chilli)
1 tsp sea salt

1. Pre-heat the oven to 180°C/350°F.

2. In a cast iron skillet or ovenproof dish, add mushrooms, melted butter, fresh thyme and garlic. Toss to coat the mushrooms in the seasonings and roast in the oven for 15 – 20 minutes until the mushrooms are soft and golden brown.

3. While the mushrooms are roasting, prepare the smash by adding avocado, cannellini beans, lemon juice, parsley, chilli flakes and sea salt into a mixing bowl. Use the back of a fork to roughly smash the ingredients together without turning it into a puree, you still want to retain some texture.

4. Remove mushrooms from the oven and pile onto a plate, spooning any pan juices over the top. Heap the avocado and white bean mash over the top and add additional seasoning if desired.

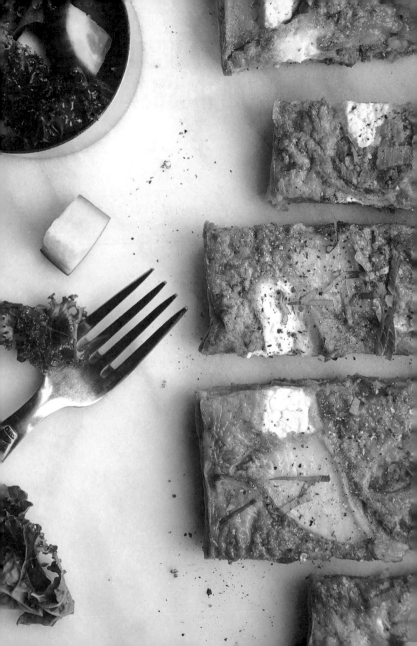

ROASTED VEGETABLE FRITTATA

Serves 4

8 eggs
½ cup (125ml) pouring cream
½ cup (50g) cheddar cheese, shredded
Sea salt and black pepper
2 cups (200g) roasted vegetables, e.g. pumpkin, potato, carrot

½ cup (100g) soft goat's cheese
Smoked paprika

1. Line a baking dish or deep tray with baking paper and preheat the oven to 200°C/390°F.

2. In a medium bowl whisk eggs with pouring cream then stir through the shredded cheese and season with salt and pepper.

3. Use leftover roast vegetables or roast some fresh for this recipe. Cut vegetables into small chunks.

4. Pour egg mixture into the lined baking pan and drop roasted vegetables evenly around the mixture. Top with small chunks of soft goat's cheese and a sprinkling of smoked paprika.

5. Bake the frittata in the oven for 30 minutes or until the egg is just set. Serve with a side of leafy greens to kick-start your day, or on its own.

one pan breakfast

Serves 1

100g/4oz haloumi cheese
2 eggs
Sea salt and black pepper
½ tsp ground cumin

1 cup (60g) kale leaves,
    chopped (stem discarded)
½ cup (40g) good quality
    sauerkraut

1. In a pan over medium heat, cook the haloumi until golden on both sides. Remove the haloumi and set aside, return pan to heat and add a drizzle of olive oil.

2. In a small bowl whisk eggs with a pinch of sea salt, black pepper and cumin.

3. Pour the egg mixture into the pan and whisk to begin scrambling.

4. After 1 minute add the chopped kale and sauerkraut and heat through for a further 1 minute.

5. Return the haloumi to the pan for the final minute of cooking before serving.

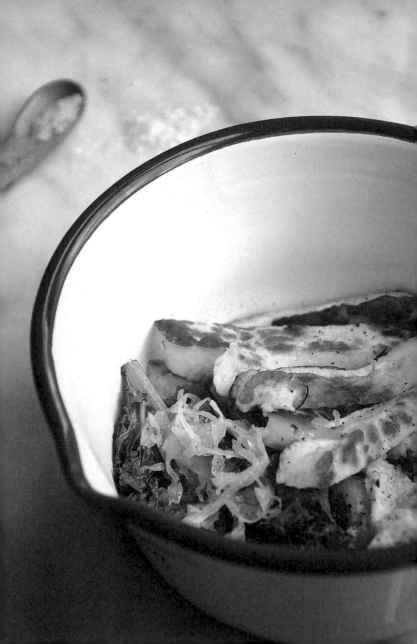

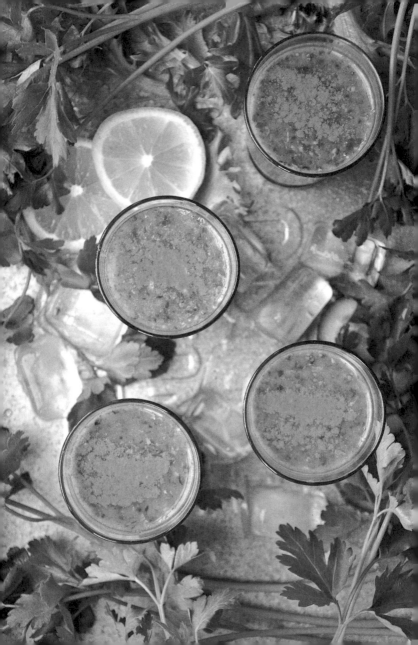

wake me up smoothie

Serves 2

1 cup (30g) baby spinach
(or kale, silver beet)
1 ripe banana (frozen
for extra creaminess)
½ an avocado
1 small cucumber
½ inch piece of fresh
ginger root

Handful of fresh parsley
1½ cups (375ml) water
¼ cup (60ml) lemon juice
(fresh)
Handful of ice
Ground turmeric for dusting

1. Chop all ingredients up into similar sized chunks.

2. Combine spinach, banana, avocado, cucumber, ginger, parsley, water, lemon juice and ice in a blender and blend on high until smooth and creamy.

3. If more liquid is needed add in additional water a little at a time until desired consistency is reached.

4. Pour into two glasses and top each with a dusting of ground turmeric. Alternatively, add the ground turmeric or a 1 inch piece of fresh turmeric at step #2.

sweet potato and bacon mini loaves

Serves 2

1 cup (150g) wholemeal
   spelt flour
½ tsp baking soda
2 tsp cinnamon
3 eggs
½ cup (125ml) coconut oil,
   melted

1 medium sweet potato
1 small zucchini (courgette)
1 tsp sea salt
1 tsp black pepper
2 bacon rashers, any cut

1. Preheat the oven to 180°C/350°F.

2. Sift flour, baking powder and cinnamon into a bowl, set aside.

3. Whisk eggs and coconut oil together and fold through the dry mixture.

4. Grate the sweet potato and zucchini, season with salt and pepper and add to the mixture.

5. Divide the batter between two mini loaf pans. Alternatively, use one larger loaf pan and increase the cooking time.

6. Dice bacon and sprinkle evenly over the top of each loaf.

7. Bake in the oven for 50 – 60 minutes. Test it is cooked through when an inserted skewer comes out clean.

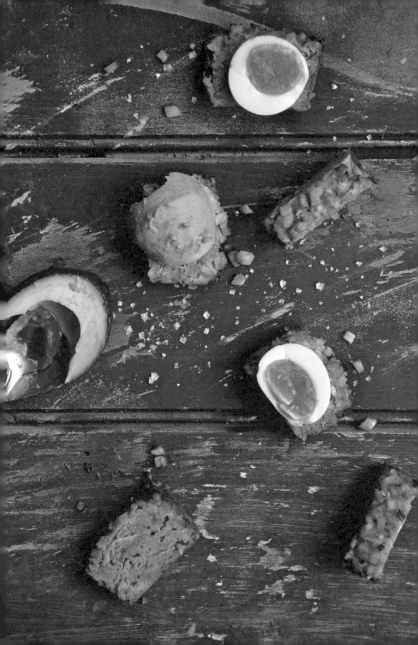

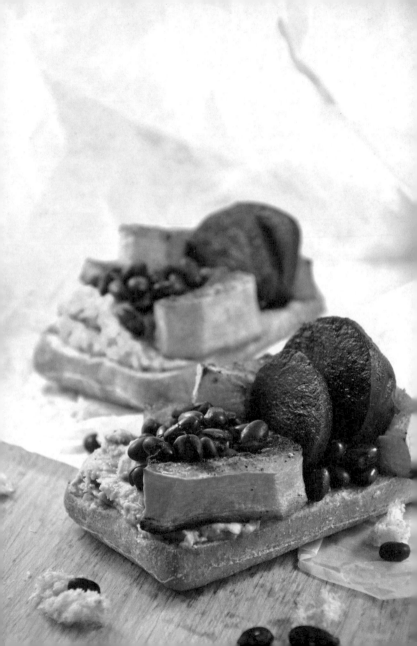

CHUNKY VEG BRUSCHETTA

Serves 2

250g/9oz pumpkin, any variety
Extra virgin olive oil
1 tsp chilli flakes
    or ground paprika
1 avocado
Sea salt

Juice of ½ lemon
2 cooked beetroot, sliced
1 cup (200g) cooked
    black beans
2 slices of your choice of bread
    or baguette

1. Preheat the oven to 180°C/350°F and line an oven tray with baking paper.

2. Cut the pumpkin into crescents or chunks, place on tray and drizzle over olive oil. Season with sea salt and chilli flakes or ground paprika. Roast in the oven for 30 minutes or until tender. This can be prepared the night before and stored in the refrigerator.

3. Prepare the guacamole by mashing or pureeing avocado, sea salt and lemon juice together.

4. Warm beans up in a small pan if desired or serve at room temperature.

5. Toast bread, spread each slice with guacamole and top with roasted pumpkin, beetroot and beans.

LUNCH

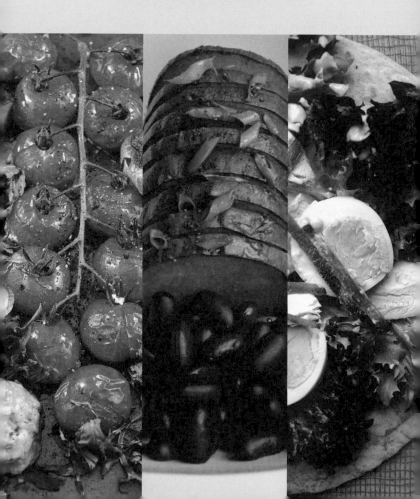

BLAT PLATTER

HASSLEBACK SWEET POTATOES
WITH CREAMED SPINACH

BAKED FALAFEL & CUCUMBER
SALAD WITH PEPITA CRUMBLE

ROAST CHICKEN
CAESAR SALAD WRAPS

MINESTRONE SOUP

SIMPLE TUNA SALAD

ROASTED TOMATO, EGGPLANT
AND CHICKPEA SALAD

BLAT PLATTER

Serves 2

12 cherry tomatoes
4 bacon rashers, any cut
1 large avocado
Handful of fresh coriander,
    use the leaves and stem

Juice of ½ lemon
Pinch of sea salt
200g/7oz baby kale leaves
Olive oil spray

1. Preheat the oven to 180°C/350°F.

2. Place cherry tomatoes on a tray, spray with olive oil and sprinkle over a pinch of sea salt and freshly ground black pepper. Roast in the oven for 20 minutes until the tomatoes are soft and begin bursting from their skins.

3. Once you have removed the tomatoes from the oven, turn the temperature up to 200°C/390°F. Curl bacon rashers into rosettes and place each inside the hole of a muffin tin. Bake the bacon in the oven for 15 - 20 minutes.

4. While the bacon is cooking, prepare the guacamole by removing the avocado flesh from the skin and blitzing in a food processor or with a hand blender, along with the coriander, lemon juice and sea salt.

5. When the bacon has 5 minutes remaining, spread the baby kale over an oven tray and spray lightly with olive oil. Bake for 3 – 5 minutes until just beginning to crisp up, careful not to let it burn.

6. Plate up the platter by layering baby kale with tomatoes and bacon and spooning or using a piping bag to pipe guacamole around the dish. Serve with crusty bread.

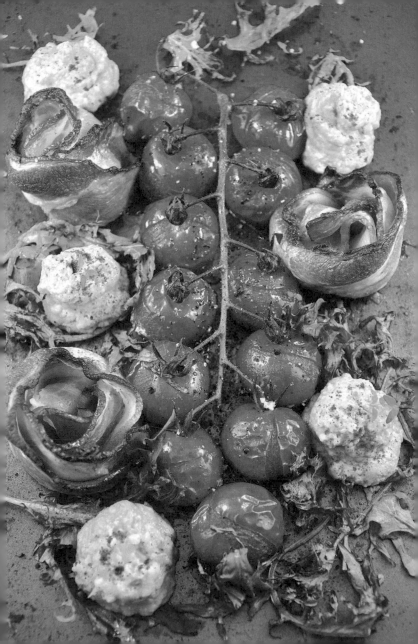

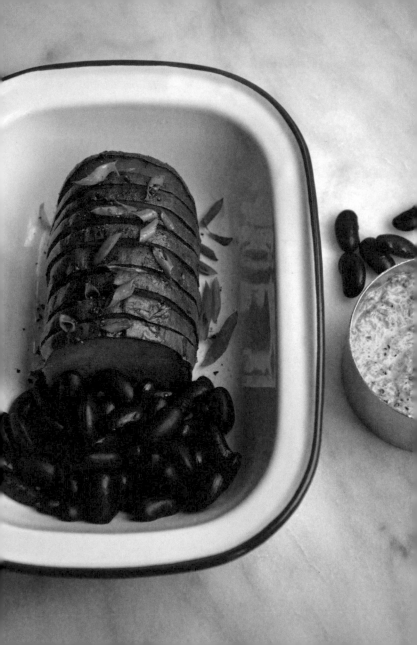

HASSLEBACK SWEET POTATOES WITH CREAMED SPINACH

Serves 2

1 large sweet potato
200g/7oz baby spinach leaves
1 tbsp chives,
   roughly chopped
Coconut milk

1 cup (150g) kidney beans
2 garlic cloves, minced
Spring onions (scallions)
   for serving
Sea salt and black pepper

1. Preheat the oven to 180°C/350°F.

2. Cut slits 2/3 way through the sweet potato and place in an oven dish or deep pan. Drizzle with olive oil and season with sea salt and black pepper. Bake for 30 – 40 minutes or until tender.

3. Prepare creamed spinach by blitzing baby spinach and chives with a pinch of sea salt. Pour coconut milk in a little at a time to reach desired consistency, amount will vary depending on how thick or runny you like it. Heat creamed spinach up in a small saucepan directly before serving.

4. Warm kidney beans up in a small pan with a drizzle of olive oil and the minced garlic for 3 – 5 minutes.

5. Divide sweet potato in half and serve with kidney beans, creamed spinach and a side salad if desired.

Baked Falafel & Cucumber Salad with Pepita Crumble

Serves 2

1 brown onion, peeled
   and quartered
1½ cups (400g) cooked
   chickpeas
2 tsp ground cumin
2 tsp ground coriander
½ cup (20g) fresh coriander
2 tbsp extra virgin olive oil
2 tbsp almond meal

1 tsp sea salt
1 large cucumber,
   any variety
1 tbsp sumac
⅔ cup (120g) pepitas
   (pumpkin seeds)
1 tbsp coconut oil, melted
1 tsp chilli flakes
Pinch of sea salt

1. Preheat the oven to 180°C/350°F.

2. In the bowl of a food processor combine onion, chickpeas, cumin, coriander, almond meal and extra virgin olive oil. Blitz until a chunky paste forms.

3. Line an oven tray with baking paper and roll spoonfuls of the falafel mix into balls in your hands. Evenly space the balls on the tray and bake in the oven for 15 – 20 minutes.

4. Dice the cucumber and toss in the sumac, set aside.

5. Coat the pepitas in coconut oil, chilli flakes and sea salt. Heat a frying pan over a medium heat and toast the pepitas until fragrant. Transfer pepitas to the bowl of a food processor and blitz into a crumble.

6. Assemble the salad with cucumber and falafels, top with the crumble and an optional drizzle of natural yoghurt.

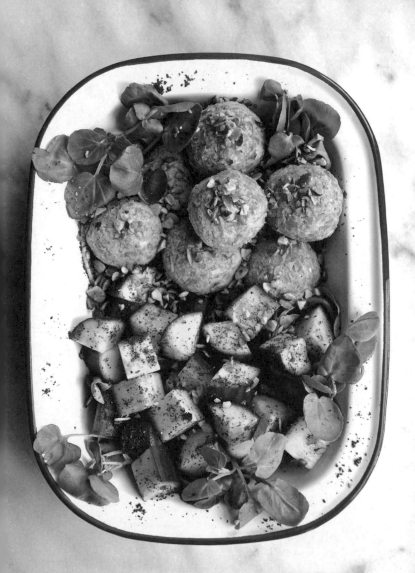

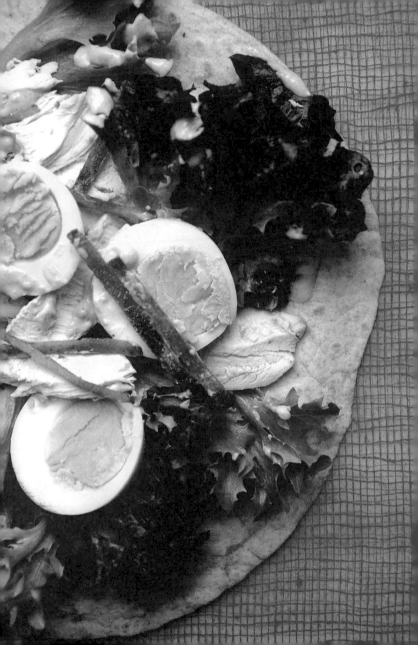

ROAST CHICKEN CAESAR SALAD WRAPS

Serves 1

1 tbsp hulled tahini
Pinch of sea salt
1 tbsp water
1 tbsp lemon juice
1 wrap of choice (e.g. rye,
    rice flour etc)
3 lettuce leaves

150g/5oz roast chicken
1 hardboiled egg, sliced
1 bacon rasher
3-4 Parmesan shavings
    (optional)

1. Prepare the tahini sauce by whisking tahini, sea salt, water and lemon juice together. Add more water as needed to reach desired consistency.

2. Spread half the sauce over the wrap and add shredded lettuce, roast chicken and egg to one side.

3. Cook the bacon in a small pan and slice into batons. Lay the bacon on top of the egg and add Parmesan shavings if using (anchovies are another filling you could include). Drizzle remaining tahini sauce over the top.

4. Roll the wrap to enclose the filling and enjoy.

MINESTRONE SOUP

Serves 6

25g/1oz butter, cubed
4 celery stalks, diced
2 medium carrots, diced
1 medium zucchini, diced
1 tbsp dried basil
1 tsp sea salt

1 tsp smoked paprika
1 tbsp tomato puree
4 cups (1L) beef stock
2 cups (500ml) water
2 cups (400g) cooked
   red kidney beans

1. In a deep saucepan melt butter and add diced celery, carrots, zucchini, dried basil, sea salt, smoked paprika and tomato puree. Stir together and sweat the vegetables for 5 minutes.

2. Add the beef stock and water and bring to a simmer, cook on a medium heat for 20 minutes until vegetables are tender and the liquid has thickened slightly. Add more water as needed during the cooking time to reach desired consistency.

3. Stir through kidney beans and heat for approximately 5 minutes before serving.

Simple Tuna Salad

Serves 1

8 cherry tomatoes
1 small cucumber, diced
½ Spanish (red) onion,
    finely sliced

150-180g/5-6oz fresh
    tuna steak
Sea salt and black pepper
Extra virgin olive oil

1. In a pan, drizzle a small amount of extra virgin olive oil and cook the cherry tomatoes for 3 – 4 minutes until the skins begin to darken and the tomatoes soften. Set aside.

2. Season both sides of the tuna with sea salt and black pepper; use your hands to press the seasoning into the flesh.

3. Heat a small pan with a drizzle of extra virgin olive oil. Gently lay the tuna steak into the hot pan and cook on low for 1 – 2 minutes each side. Remove from pan and rest for 4 minutes before slicing.

4. Assemble the salad by layering the tuna on top of the cucumber, red onion and cherry tomatoes. Drizzle a small amount of extra virgin olive oil over the top if desired.

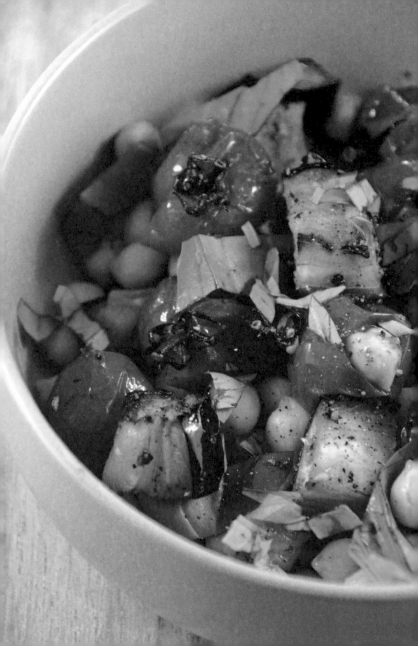

ROASTED TOMATO, EGGPLANT AND CHICKPEA SALAD

Serves 1

1 cup (140g) cherry
   or Roma tomatoes
   (or any small variety)
1 cup (100g) eggplant
   (aubergine), diced
⅓ cup (80ml) extra virgin
   olive oil
2 tsp sea salt
1 tsp black pepper

1 cup (240g) cooked
   chickpeas
⅓ cup (40g) fresh basil
   leaves, chopped
¼ cup (60ml) fresh
   lemon juice
Pinch of sea salt and
   ground black pepper

1. Preheat the oven to 180°C/350°F.

2. In a shallow baking dish, combine cherry tomatoes and eggplant with olive oil. Sprinkle over sea salt and black pepper before tossing gently. Roast in the oven for 20 – 30 minutes until the eggplant is tender and the tomatoes are bursting from their skins.

3. Remove from the oven and while still warm toss through the chickpeas, fresh basil leaves and lemon juice. Taste and adjust seasoning with additional sea salt or black pepper as needed.

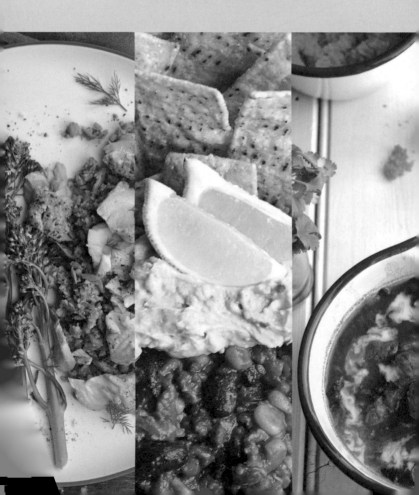

DINNER

SPICY BEEF AND SPINACH CURRY

PAN SEARED SALMON WITH
DILL PEA MASH

MEXICAN CASSEROLE
WITH CORIANDER GUACAMOLE

SPICED BROCCOLI, KALE
& LENTIL BOWLS

RED CHICKEN WITH PRESERVED
LEMON CAULIFLOWER

NAKED BEAN BURGERS

SWEET POTATO NACHOS

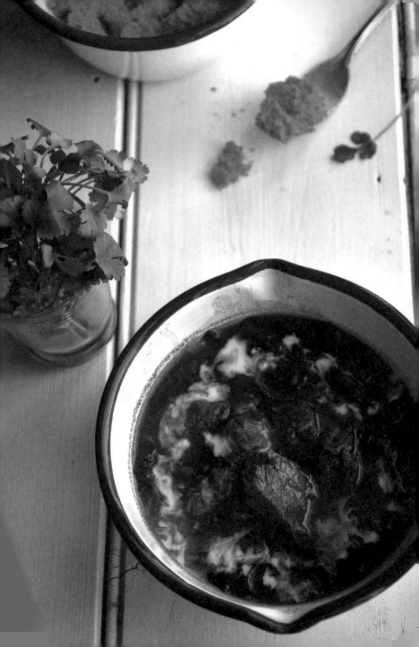

SPICY BEEF AND SPINACH CURRY

Serves 2 – 4

500g/1lb sirloin
or rump steak
½ Spanish (red) onion,
finely chopped
1 inch piece of fresh
ginger root, finely grated
4 garlic cloves, crushed
3 red chillies (any variety),
finely chopped

1 green chilli (any variety),
finely chopped
1⅔ cups (250g) diced
tomatoes
2 cups (500ml) beef stock,
plus more stock or water
as needed

1. Slice beef into thin strips and sprinkle lightly with sea salt.

2. Heat up a large cast iron pot or saucepan over a medium heat. Add a drizzle of extra virgin olive oil and add onion, ginger, garlic and chilli. Sweat for 3-5 minutes. Add the beef, tomatoes and stock, stir and reduce the heat to low.

3. Simmer for 45-60 minutes until the beef is tender, checking every 15 minutes and adding additional stock or water as needed.

4. Serve on a bed of cooked rice or mashed sweet potato, with a side of steamed green vegetables and natural yoghurt to dissipate the heat if needed.

NOTE: Adjust spice-level to your taste buds by using less chillies if necessary.

Pan Seared Salmon with Dill Pea Mash

Serves 2

2 salmon fillets
1 tsp sea salt
1 tsp black pepper
Zest of 1 lemon
Extra virgin olive oil

3 cups (385g) peas
250g/9oz broccolini
1 tbsp unsalted butter
¼ cup (25g) fresh dill,
    finely chopped

1. Season each salmon fillet with sea salt, black pepper and lemon zest. Drizzle with extra virgin olive oil and set aside.

2. Heat a frying pan over a medium heat and add the salmon skin side down. Cook for 4 minutes each side.

3. While the salmon is cooking, steam the peas and broccolini until tender then stir through the butter and dill. Set the broccolini aside and mash the peas roughly with a fork.

4. Serve the salmon fillets on top of the pea mash and alongside the broccolini. Squeeze fresh lemon juice over the top if desired.

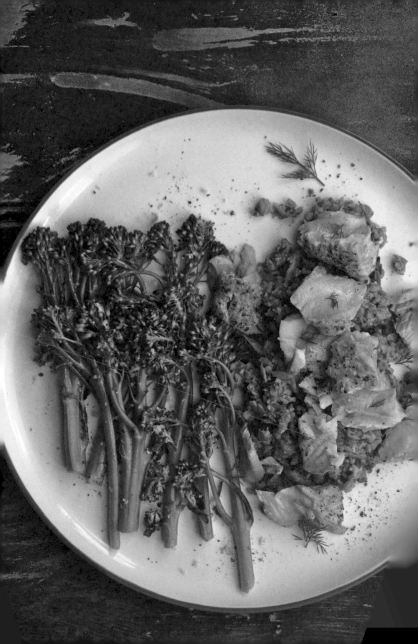

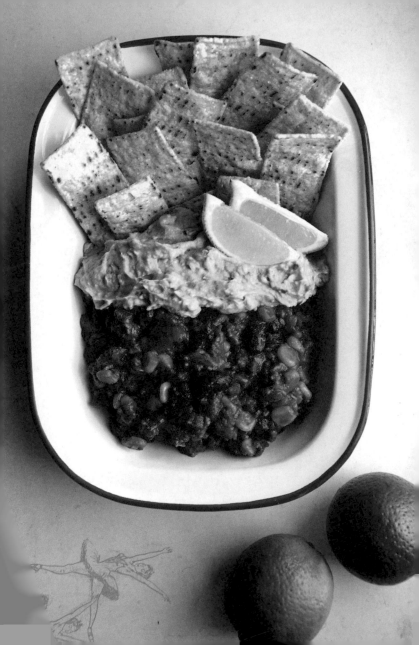

Mexican Casserole with Coriander Guacamole

Serves 4

1 brown onion, diced
2 red chillis or 1 tbsp dried red chilli
3 garlic cloves, minced
1 tbsp smoked paprika
500g/1lb beef mince
1 red capsicum (pepper), diced
1 yellow capsicum (pepper), diced

1 cup (250g) crushed tomatoes
1½ cups (300g) cooked kidney beans (or bean of choice)
1 cup (250g) corn kernels
1 avocado, any variety
½ cup (20g) coriander leaves
Juice of 1 lemon
Pinch of sea salt

1. Preheat the oven to 180°C/350°F.

2. Heat a saucepan and add a drizzle of extra virgin olive oil followed by the onion, chilli, garlic and paprika. Cook for 4 minutes before adding beef and cooking on low for 15-20 minutes.

3. Add the capsicums, kidney beans, corn and crushed tomatoes. Heat until warmed through.

4. Prepare the guacamole by mashing the avocado, coriander leaves, lemon juice and sea salt to desired consistency.

5. Serve the casserole with guacamole, extra coriander and corn chips if desired.

SPICED BROCCOLI, KALE & LENTIL BOWLS

Serves 2

½ tsp ground cumin
½ tsp chilli flakes (or fresh chilli)
¼ tsp cinnamon
¼ tsp ground coriander
¼ tsp ground fenugreek (optional)
Sea salt
1 garlic clove, crushed
1 inch piece of fresh ginger root, grated

1 head of broccoli (including stem), cut into small chunks
1½ cups (100g) kale, roughly chopped
1 can (400g/14oz) of cooked lentils
2 tbsp coconut oil
2 tbsp coconut milk
Zest of ½ lemon
¼ cup (30g) walnut pieces

1. Combine all spices in a bowl.

2. Lightly steam broccoli and kale and set aside.

3. Drain the lentils and rinse thoroughly under water.

4. In a pan over medium heat add the oil and spice mix, cooking gently to release the aromas.

5. Add the broccoli, kale and lentils and coat with the spices. Heat through.

6. Serve the spiced broccoli, kale and lentils with coconut milk, lemon zest and walnuts on top.

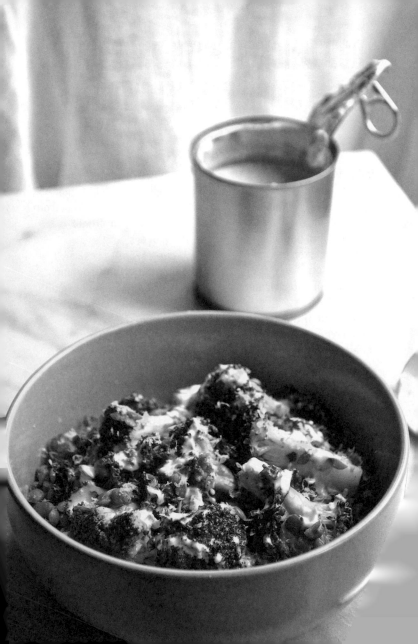

RED CHICKEN WITH PRESERVED LEMON CAULIFLOWER

Serves 4

Pinch of saffron threads
1/3 cup (80ml) warm water
4 garlic cloves, minced
2 tsp sea salt
1 tbsp ground paprika
500g/1lb chicken thigh fillets
¼ cup (60ml) extra virgin olive oil
1/3 cup (80ml) thickened (heavy) cream
1 head of cauliflower

3 small preserved lemons (approximately 1 inch diameter each) *buy from specialty or ethnic grocers
½ cup (125ml) preserved lemon brine (from jar)
2 tbsp extra virgin olive oil
2 tbsp dried rosemary
2 tsp sea salt
1 tsp black pepper

1. Preheat the oven to 180°C/356°F.

2. Add saffron threads to the warm water in a small bowl and stir. Let the saffron release its colour into the water for 10 minutes.

3. Mince the garlic and add to a medium bowl with the saffron water and threads. Stir through sea salt and paprika.

4. Cut the chicken thighs into thirds and coat in the marinade. Set aside while preparing the cauliflower.

5. Cut the head of cauliflower into florets and place in a large mixing bowl.

6. Finely slice the preserved lemons and add to the bowl with the brine, olive oil, rosemary, salt and pepper, stir until combined. Line an oven tray with baking paper and spread the cauliflower evenly out. Roast for 20 – 30 minutes until brown on top and tender.

7. While the cauliflower is roasting, heat a pan over medium heat on the stove and add the chicken thighs and any of the leftover marinade. Cook for 20 minutes, testing one piece of chicken to ensure it is cooked through.

8. Stir through the cream and cook for a further 5 minutes before removing from the heat.

9. Serve red chicken with lemon cauliflower and steamed greens on the side. Optional extras could include mashed sweet potato, lentils or steamed rice.

NOTE: If you can't source preserved lemons, try substituting with homemade lemon oil.

Remove the peel from 6 lemons, careful not to leave any flesh on them. Rinse under water and dry thoroughly with paper towel before placing in a jar and pouring over 3 cups (750ml) of good quality extra virgin olive oil.

Tightly seal the lid and store for a minimum of 2 weeks to let the flavour infuse. Use in the recipe in place of the extra virgin olive oil and the preserved lemon brine and simply coat the cauliflower lightly with the lemon oil.

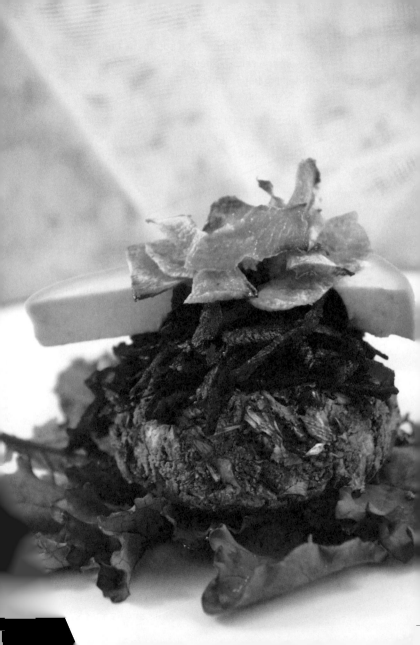

NAKED BEAN BURGERS

Serves 4

2 cups (400g) cooked
   kidney beans
2 cups (400g) cooked
   black beans
3 spring onions (scallions)
1 tsp sea salt

1 tsp black pepper
2 tsp smoked paprika
1 medium beetroot,
   raw but peeled
1 medium sweet potato
1 avocado

1. Preheat the oven to 180°C/350°F.

2. In the bowl of a food processor combine the kidney beans and black beans. Slice spring onions and stir through the bean mixture with sea salt, black pepper and smoked paprika. Divide the mixture into 4 portions and roll each into a hamburger-shaped patty. Place each patty on a baking paper-lined tray and bake in the oven for 20 minutes, set aside to cool before removing from the tray.

3. Grate the beetroot using a box cutter or food processor. Slice avocado and drizzle lemon juice over the top to stop the avocado browning.

4. To make the sweet potato crisps, use a vegetable peeler to peel thin slices or chip off little crisp-size bites. Lay the sweet potato on an oven tray lined with baking paper. Drizzle extra virgin olive oil over the top and sprinkle with a pinch of sea salt. Bake in the oven for 10 – 15 minutes or until crisp.

5. Assemble the burger by placing the patty on a small pile of baby kale or lettuce leaves, top with avocado and the raw shredded beetroot. Sprinkle the sweet potato chips over the top.

sweet potato nachos

Serves 2

2 medium sweet potatoes
Olive oil spray
1 tsp smoked paprika
1 cup (180g) cooked kidney
or black beans
2 garlic cloves, minced

1 medium red capsicum
(pepper)
1 small Spanish (red) onion
1 large avocado
Juice of ½ lemon
Handful of coriander leaves

1. Preheat the oven to 200°C/390°F and line an oven tray with baking paper.

2. Using a knife or mandolin, slice the sweet potatoes into thin rounds and place in a single layer on the oven tray. Spray with olive oil and sprinkle the smoked paprika over the top. Season with sea salt and black pepper if desired.Bake the chips in the oven for 20 – 30 minutes; keep an eye on them so they don't burn.

3. While the chips are cooking prepare the guacamole by blitzing the avocado, lemon juice and coriander in a food processor, using a stick blender or mashing with a fork for a chunkier texture. Season with sea salt and black pepper.

4. Thoroughly rinse the cooked beans. In a small pan over a low heat, add a drizzle of olive oil, the beans and the minced garlic until heated through and fragrant.

5. Thinly slice the capsicum and Spanish onion.

6. Construct your nachos beginning with the beans on the base and layering sweet potato, capsicum, onion and guacamole. Add additional coriander for garnish.

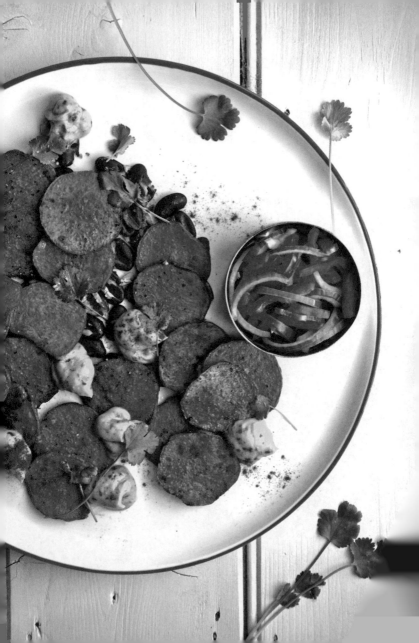

TREATS

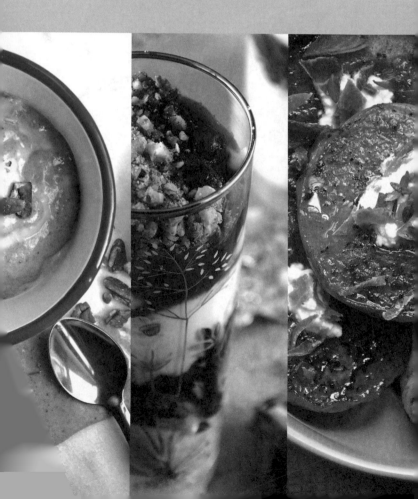

MACADAMIA ROCK CAKES

DOUBLE NUT CRUNCHES

BAKED APPLE PIE SMOOTHIE

ICED CHAI TEA

BANANA WHIP
WITH STICKY DATE SAUCE

SOUR CRANBERRY
& GINGER CRUNCH CHEESECAKE

PEACHES WITH GOAT'S CHEESE
AND CRISPY PANCETTA

CHERRY AND SEA SALT BROWNIES

PINA COLADA PLATT

Macadamia Rock Cakes

Makes 6

1½ cups (225g) macadamia
    nuts
1 cup (80g) shredded
    coconut
3 tbsp coconut butter
1 tsp sea salt
¼ cup (60ml) rice malt syrup

¼ cup (60ml) coconut oil,
    melted
¼ cup (30g) raw cacao
    powder
Pinch of sea salt
1 tbsp rice malt syrup

1. Process macadamia nuts in a food processor until crumbs form. Add the coconut, coconut butter, salt and rice malt syrup and pulse until combined.

2. Press spoonfuls of the mixture into 6 holes of a muffin tin. Keep adding mixture in until it is all used, press down hard.

3. Place tin in the refrigerator for 1 hour until the cakes have firmed up.

4. Prepare the chocolate topping by combining the coconut oil, raw cacao, sea salt and rice malt syrup. Stir until smooth.

5. Take the rock cakes out of the refrigerator and use a butter knife to help ease them out of the tin.

6. Dip the top of each cake into the chocolate mixture and turn to drain the excess. Place on a plate ready to eat or store in the refrigerator.

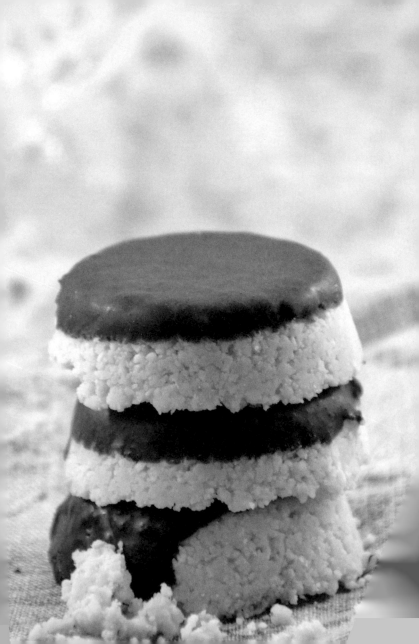

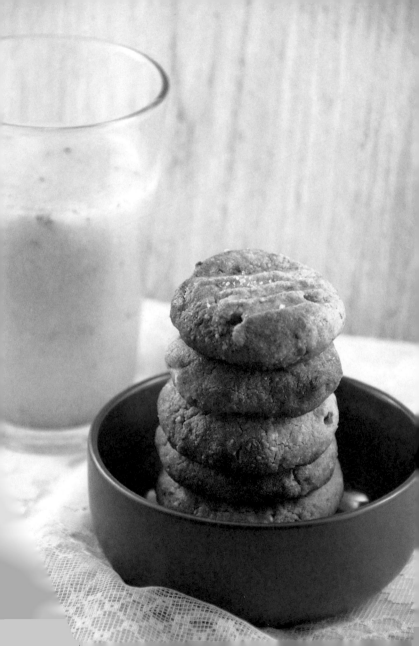

DOUBLE NUT CRUNCHES

Makes 16

1 cup (135g) smooth
   peanut butter (or other
   nut butter)
1 egg

⅓ cup (80ml) rice malt syrup
⅔ cup (80g) crushed walnuts
1 tsp ground cinnamon
Sea salt

1. Preheat the oven to 180°C/350°F.

2. In a bowl stir peanut butter, egg, rice malt syrup, walnuts and cinnamon together.

3. Take spoonfuls of the mixture and roll into balls.

4. Place on an oven tray lined with baking paper and press down with a fork. Sprinkle the tops of each cookie with a pinch of sea salt.

5. Bake in the oven for 10 minutes.

Baked Apple Pie Smoothie

Serves 1 - 2

1 medium apple, any variety
1 tsp ground cinnamon
½ tsp ground ginger
½ tsp ground nutmeg
Pinch of vanilla powder

1 tbsp coconut oil, melted
1 cup (250ml) milk of choice
   (almond, rice, full fat dairy)
4 ice cubes

1. Preheat the oven to 180°C/350°F.

2. Combine all spices in a small bowl and set aside.

3. Core the apple and lightly coat the skin with melted coconut oil using a pastry brush or by rolling the apple in the oil.

4. Roll the apple in the prepared spice mix until coated thoroughly. Place the apple on an oven tray lined with parchment paper.

5. Bake in the oven for 20 minutes or until the skin starts to crinkle and the flesh softens. Remove from the oven and set aside to cool slightly.

6. Add the apple, ice cubes and any leftover spices to a blender or use a stick mixer to process it with your milk of choice.

ICED CHAI TEA

Serves 2-4

1 chai tea bag
3 - 4 cups (750ml-1L) water
Peel of 1 lemon
¼ cup (60ml) rice malt syrup

Extra ice to serve
Water, soda water
   or almond milk

1. In a small saucepan place tea bag, water and lemon peel and bring to the boil.

2. Reduce to a simmer, remove the tea bags using tongs or a slotted spoon and stir through the rice malt syrup to desired sweetness.

3. Take off the heat and let cool to room temperature before pouring into a jar or jug and chilling in the refrigerator for at least 30 minutes.

4. To serve, fill each glass with ice cubes, pour over the tea mixture to half way up the glass and top with water, soda water, almond milk or the milk of your choice.

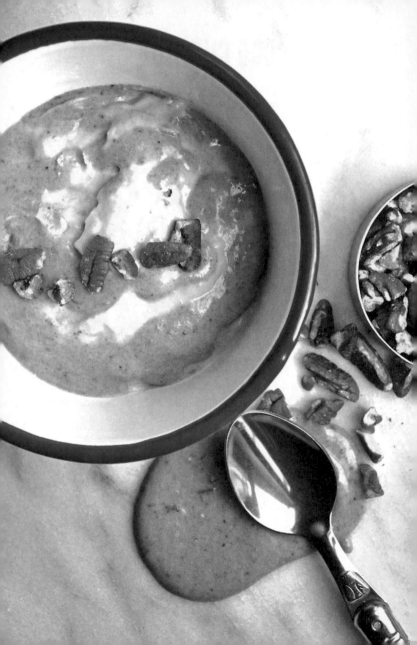

BANANA WHIP
WITH STICKY DATE SAUCE

Serves 2

2 bananas
½ cup (125ml) coconut milk
1 tsp vanilla powder
3 fresh dates, pitted
½ cup (125ml) coconut milk
Handful of pecans to serve

1. Remove the banana skins and place bananas in a plastic zip lock bag. Freeze for 1 hour.

2. Remove the bananas from the freezer and add to a blender or food processor with the coconut milk and vanilla powder. Blend until smooth and creamy.

3. Prepare the sticky date sauce by blitzing dates in a food processor and adding coconut milk a little at a time until desired consistency is reached.

4. Scoop banana whip into a bowl and pour over the sticky date sauce. You can gently heat the sauce in a small pan beforehand to turn this dessert into a winter warmer, or add toppings such as toasted coconut flakes or crushed pecans.

SOUR CRANBERRY & GINGER CRUNCH CHEESECAKE

Serves 4

250g/9oz cream cheese, at room temperature
½ cup (125ml) thickened cream
3 tbsp rice malt syrup or maple syrup
¼ cup (60ml) fresh lemon juice
1½ cups (110g) frozen cranberries (or other berry)

1 inch piece of fresh ginger, grated

GINGER CRUNCH
¼ cup (25g) quinoa flakes
¼ cup (30g) pecans
1 tbsp rice malt syrup
1 tsp ground ginger
½ tsp ground cinnamon

1. Preheat the oven to 180°C/350°F.

2. Combine cream cheese, cream, rice malt syrup and lemon juice in a food processor and blend until smooth.

3. In a small saucepan over low heat, add cranberries and fresh ginger. Cook until cranberries are soft and have released some juice. Set aside.

4. For the ginger crunch, combine quinoa flakes, pecans, rice malt syrup, ground ginger and cinnamon. Cook in the oven for 5 – 10 minutes until golden and crunchy.

5. Assemble the cheesecake in glasses or bowls, layering the cream cheese mix and cranberries until you fill the vessel. Top with the ginger crunch.

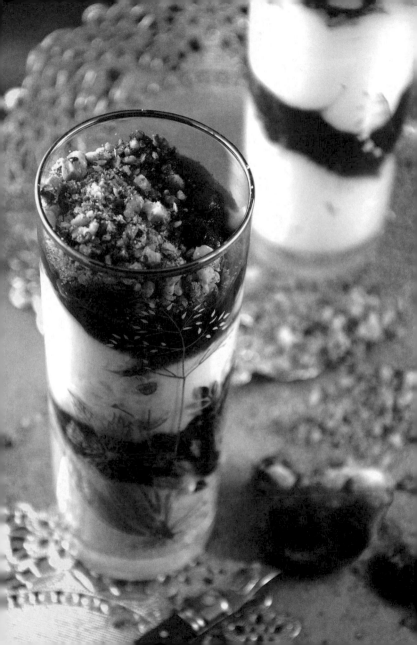

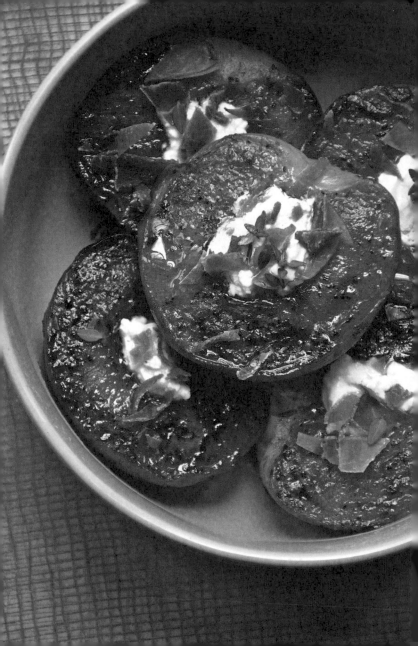

PEACHES WITH GOAT'S CHEESE AND CRISPY PANCETTA

Serves 2

25g/1oz butter, cubed
2 peaches (any variety)
½ tsp cinnamon
½ tsp nutmeg

½ tsp ground cardamom
½ tsp ground ginger
50g/2oz soft goat's cheese
2-4 thin slices of prosciutto

1. Preheat the oven to 180°C/350°F.

2. Slice peaches in half and remove pits. Heat up a cast iron skillet or a regular frying pan over a medium heat. Add the butter followed by the peaches, skin side down.

3. Mix spices together in a small bowl and then sprinkle evenly over the peaches while they're cooking.

4. Cook for 5 minutes each side until the flesh begins to soften. Meanwhile heat a small frying pan and cook the prosciutto until crisp.

5. Remove peaches from the pan, spoon goat's cheese into each peach and top with the pancetta.

CHERRY AND SEA SALT BROWNIES

Makes 12 squares

150g/5oz butter, melted
½ cup (50g) raw cacao
Pinch of vanilla powder
3 eggs
½ cup (55g) almond flour

1 cup (110g) fresh or frozen
   cherries, pitted
50-75g/2-3oz dark chocolate
   (70%+ cocoa)
2 tsp sea salt

1. Preheat the oven to 160°C/320°F.

2. In a bowl combine melted butter with cacao and vanilla powder. Stir until smooth with no lumps. Beat in eggs one at a time then fold through the almond flour. Fold through half the cherries, reserving the remaining half for the top of the brownies.

3. Roughly chop the dark chocolate, add half to the brownie batter and reserve half to top the brownies with. Sprinkle 1 teaspoon of the sea salt into the batter and stir to combine.

4. Pour the batter into a brownie or baking tin lined with greaseproof paper. If you're wanting tall brownies, opt for a smaller tin with higher walls, or use a flatter, longer tin for thinner treats.

5. Smooth the top of the mixture in the tin and dot the surface with remaining cherries and dark chocolate. Sprinkle the remaining teaspoon of sea salt evenly over the top of the brownie.

6. Bake in the oven for 25-30 minutes until an inserted skewer comes out clean.

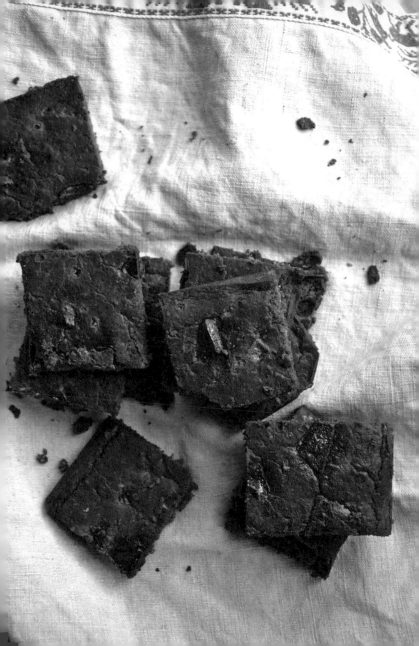

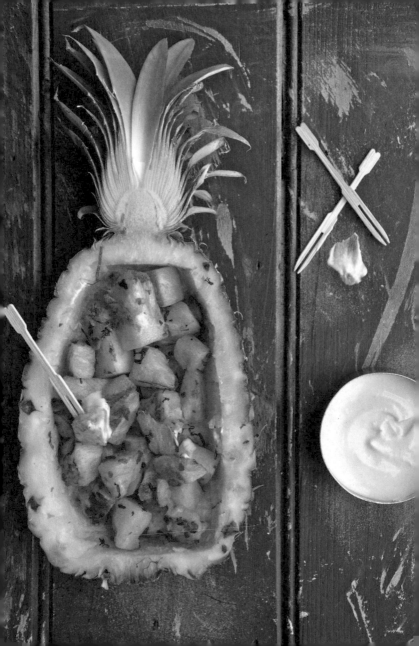

PINA COLADA PLATTER

Serves 2

½ large fresh pineapple
¼ cup (60ml) coconut oil,
　melted
1-2 tbsp chilli (red pepper)
　flakes
1 tsp sea salt

DIPPING SAUCE
1 cup (250ml) coconut milk
Handful of fresh mint leaves,
　finely sliced

1. The night before serving this dessert, place the coconut milk for the dipping sauce in the refrigerator.

2. Remove the skin from the pineapple and cut the flesh into chunks. In a medium bowl, combine melted coconut oil with chilli flakes and sea salt. Add the pineapple and toss to coat.

3. Heat up a skillet or frying pan and cook pineapple for 5-10 minutes until golden on the outside.

4. Meanwhile prepare the dipping sauce by removing the coconut milk from the refrigerator and whisking it for 3-5 minutes to help thicken it up. You can add a pinch of vanilla powder if you like or leave it plain.

5. Transfer the pineapple from the skillet to a serving platter and scatter finely chopped mint over the top. Alternatively, you can serve the pineapple chunks in the hollowed out pineapple for a party, and make sure to provide toothpicks or small skewers for guests to pick up and dip the pineapple with.

TALK THE TALK WHILE YOU WALK THE WALK

Positive language concerning food and eating habits is vital to sticking to a healthy lifestyle, which means negativity is strictly forbidden. Even if you feel positive in mind and spirit, all it takes is one friend having a bad day, or one overly opinionated family member or co-worker to derail you.

While the common diet (designed to fail), relies on you breaking the rules and feeling shame, embarrassment and even self loathing, when changing your lifestyle and lowering your sugar intake it's these "failures" that will make you stronger in the long run. It's the moments you slip, overindulge or make the less desirable choice that will cement for you how your body works on low sugar and how it feels when you fall back on old habits.

Talking your health and your choices down is a great way to fast track self-loathing and won't make achieving your health goals any easier. Remember: what you used to eat is in the past and cannot be changed, what you might eat in the future is not worth your time worrying about, but what you feed your body at this exact moment is completely in your control.

Above all, you are not what you eat, you are a complex and beautiful person and each day offers another opportunity to learn and grow.

You've come so far in 30 days; don't let these phrases come out of your mouth:

✗ I can't eat that.
✗ I'm not allowed to eat that.
✗ I wish I could eat that.
✗ You're so lucky you get to eat that.
✗ I'd kill for some chocolate.
✗ I just ate some chocolate, I feel terrible.
✗ I've failed.
✗ I cheated.
✗ I couldn't even last a week, I'm pathetic.
✗ I should be doing better by now.

Replace negative talk with affirmations:
✔ I choose to eat this.
✔ I choose not to eat that.
✔ I hit a bump in the road but tomorrow is a new day.
✔ I am more than what I eat.
✔ I'm doing so well.
✔ Today I am happy, healthy and in control of my life
✔ What can I learn from this?

You are not what you eat, you are a complex and beautiful person and each day offers another opportunity to learn and grow.